HAYFA BERGAOUI
YESSINE BELHAJTAHER
IMEN GHADHAB

Management of elderly primiparous women: PREGNANCY AND DELIVERY

HAYFA BERGAOUI
YESSINE BELHAJTAHER
IMEN GHADHAB

Management of elderly primiparous women: PREGNANCY AND DELIVERY

ScienciaScripts

Cover image: www.ingimage.com

This book is a translation from the original published under ISBN 978-620-6-71208-4.

Publisher:
Sciencia Scripts
is a trademark of
Dodo Books Indian Ocean Ltd. and OmniScriptum S.R.L publishing group

120 High Road, East Finchley, London, N2 9ED, United Kingdom
Str. Armeneasca 28/1, office 1, Chisinau MD-2012, Republic of Moldova, Europe
Printed at: see last page
ISBN: 978-620-8-08161-4

Contents

1 Introduction

Pregnancy-related complications are one of the world's major public health problems. According to data from the World Health Organisation (WHO), in 2015, more than 300,000 women died during the gravidopuerperal period. Despite considerable efforts to reduce maternal mortality, almost 800 women die every day from complications related to pregnancy or childbirth, and around 99% of these deaths occur in low- and middle-income countries (1).

Late pregnancies are a hot topic for women and perinatal health professionals alike.

In 1958, FIGO (Federation Internationale de Gynecologie Obstetrique) defined late pregnancies as pregnancies occurring after the age of 35.

In our context, women over 35 are considered to be of advanced obstetrical age(2).

the age of 35 is the most frequently used age for primiparous women (3).

However, certain complications may arise during pregnancy and/or delivery. These complications are all the more frequent when the pregnant woman is very young or old (3).

Pregnancy in older primiparous women has long been of concern to obstetricians, because it involves risks associated with the first delivery and risks associated with age (3). In fact, the literature as a whole recognises that advanced maternal age is a risk factor in the etiology of a number of pregnancy-related pathologies.

These late pregnancies occur in a variety of circumstances:

- the use of safe contraception to control fertility means that couples can now plan their pregnancies.
- the progress of medically assisted procreation, which attempts to fulfil the desire for pregnancy at any age.
- the late start, long studies, the importance attached to professional careers, and a second union with a desire to have children with the new partner.

Whereas in the past, the birth of a child at an advanced age most often corresponded to the arrival of the youngest child in a large sibling group, today we see more and more women becoming mothers for the first time aged 40 and over.

This raises the question, for the professionals involved, of the impact of age on pregnancy on the one hand, and the possible need to adapt conventional pregnancy monitoring to the characteristics of this population of older pregnant women on the other.

In this work, we aim to demonstrate the interest and benefits of describing the management of elderly primiparous women in terms of short- and long-term improvement in maternal-fetal prognosis:

- Describing the maternal-fetal complications of advanced pregnancy.
- -Describing the role of the midwife in caring for elderly parturients.

Finally, let's not forget that a better understanding of this phenomenon would enable us to answer these women's questions about the risks of motherhood.

2 Materials and methods

I. Type of study :

In order to achieve our objectives, we carried out a retrospective study in 2021/2022 of 50 cases of elderly primiparous women.

Information on these cases will be provided by the medical files in the Gynecology-Obstetrics Department of the Monastir Maternity and Neonatology Centre.

II. Sample criteria

- Inclusion criteria:

parturients included in this study must meet the following criteria:

-primiparous

-age >38

- 1 exclusion criteria :

-multiparous

-age <38

III. Parameters collected

- For data collection, we use the medical and obstetrical records of the Gynecology-Obstetrics Department of the Monastir Maternity and Neonatology Centre.
- Maternity ward and delivery registers

A data collection form has been filled in for each parturient, containing the following information

1-maternal characteristics :

- Age
- Family situation
- Profession
- Consumption of toxic substances
- BMI
- Gestite / parite
- History of: abortion/arrested pregnancy/EPU/
- Maternal pathologies

2-About the pregnancy studied :

- number of prenatal consultations
- Getting pregnant: spontaneously or with the help of MAP
- wanted / unplanned pregnancy
- type of pregnancy: mono-final/multiple

3-pathologies of pregnancy :

- maternal pathology(ies) :

- PAD /HTA gravidarum/ TG / Eclampsia
- GD/thyroid disease/other
- LA pathologies
- final pathologies :

- chromosomal malformations/anomalies

-IUGR / macrosomia / IUGR / other

4-Screening for trisomy 21 :

-Triple test

-Amniocentese

-No screening

5-The work process:

- The term
- Total working hours
- The start of work spt / declenche
- Rupture of the water sac:

spt/artificial

- Analgesia/no analgesia
- With Syntocinon /Without Syntocinon
- Streptococcus screening B :

done/not done

6-Giving birth:

-AVB

-Instrumental extractions

-With perineal lesions / without perineal lesions

-C/S

-Delivery : spt /directed / artificial

7-The condition of the child at birth :

-Weight/Colour of amniotic fluid

-APGAR

- Prematurity / IUGR / Neonatal mortality / others -Neonatal transfer

8-Following childbirth:

-Breastfeeding : Maternal / Artificial

-PP pathologies: PP hemorrhage/MTE/other

- Length of stay

IV. Statistical study

The data was entered and analysed using SPSS software.

V.Ethics :

Our work does not pose any ethical problems, as the proposed study poses no danger to the patient. The patient's anonymity and the confidentiality of information are respected when accessing the file. Our study complies with the requirements of the ethics committee and has been authorised by the head of the maternity department.

3 Results

I. Epidemiology

1. Frequency

During the study period, we recorded 50 observations of primiparous women aged over 38 who gave birth at the Monastir maternity hospital, representing 0.58% of deliveries.

2. Age distribution

the maximum frequency in older primiparous women is at the age of 38

The average age was 40, ranging from 38 to 47.

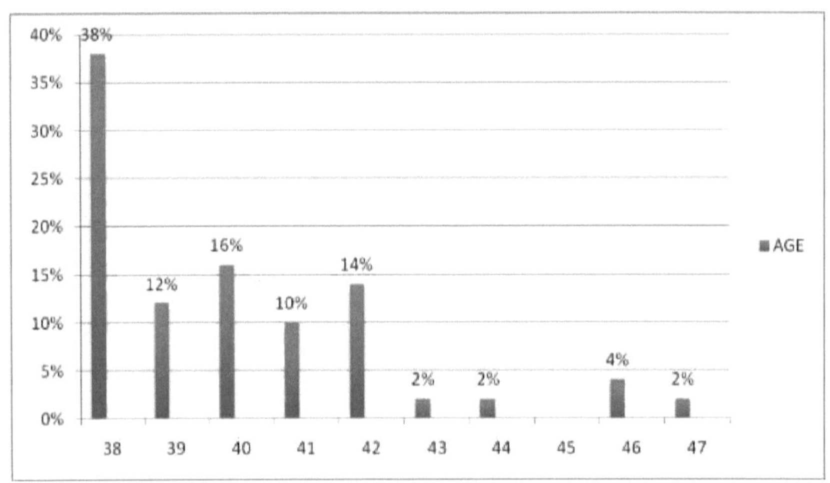

Figure 1 Frequency of age in older primiparas

3. Breakdown by occupation

Most older first-time mothers are workers.

62% of <u>older first-time mothers were in work</u>

Percentage	
No profession	38%
Worker	48%
Middle management	4%
Senior executive	10%

Table 1 Occupational activity of older primiparous women

4. Height and weight of old primiparous cows

4.1. Size

The average height of our old primiparous dams is 160.24 cm, with extremes ranging from 146 cm to 174 cm.

4.2. Weight

The average weight of our parturients ranged from 60kg to 148kg, with an average of 82kg, and 54% were obese women.

	ICM	Number	%
Normal woman	18-25	2	4%
Overweight	25-30	21	42%
Obeses	>30	27	54%

Table 2 Distribution according to ICM

II. CAUSES Causes of late-onset primiparitis

Causes	Numbers	Percentages
Late marriage	**13**	**26%**
Sterility	**7**	**14%**
Abortions	**4**	**8%**
Late marriage +sterilitis	**9**	**18%**
Late marriage + Abortion	**17**	**34%**

Table 3 causes of late-onset primiparity

1. Late marriage

Women's involvement in further education and professional activities are the most likely to be essential.

2. Abortions

Twenty-one primiparous women had one or more miscarriages, i.e. between 42% and 58% of women were primigravida at the time of delivery.

First gesture	**56%**
Second gesture	30%
Third gesture	4%

Fourth gesture	8%
Fifth gesture	0%
Sixth gesture	0%
Seventh gesture	2%

Table 4 Percentage of gestite at delivery

3. Infertility

- Only 8 pregnancies were obtained by MAP, while infertility was found in 16 cases.
- 6 elderly primiparous mothers had infertility for more than 10 years
- Our study did not identify the male or female causes of infertility because we did not have all the reports at the time of data collection.

4. Other causes

The change of spouse appears to be a cause of late procreation, and this factor could not be studied in our retrospective work due to a lack of information on the files.

III. Pathologies prior to the current pregnancy

1. Medical conditions

Pathologies	Numbers	Percentages
Hypertension	**1**	**2%**
Diabetes	**2**	**4%**
Hepatitis B	**3**	**6%**
Asthma	**3**	**6%**
Other	**2**	**4%**

Table 5 Breakdown of patients by medical history

2. Surgical pathologies

9 elderly primiparous dams (18%) underwent surgery

Intervention	Number	Percentage
Surgical treatment of ovarian cyst 1	**3**	**6%**

Myomectomies	**3**	**6%**
Surgical treatment of hydatid cysts in the liver	**1**	**2%**
Other surgeries	**2**	**4%**

Table 6: Surgical history of elderly primiparous women

3. Gyneco-obstetric diseases

Pathologies	Numbers	Percentage
Fibroids	4	8%
Ovarian cyst	3	6%
Abortions	21	42%
Voluntary termination of pregnancy	0	0%
Other	3	6%

Table 7: gynaecological-obstetric antecedents in primiparous aged women

IV. course of the pregnancy

1. Pregnancy fashion

Most pregnancies are spontaneous

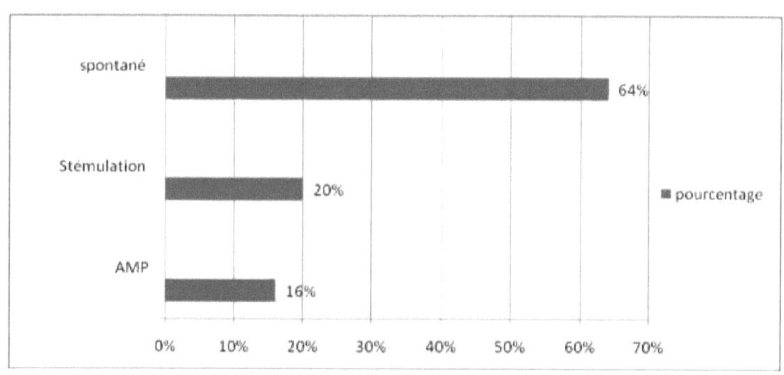

Figure 2: mode of pregnancy

	Number	Percentage
ANC >5	46	92%
CPN<5	4	8%
Total	50	100%

Table 8: Pregnancy follow-up

- Gestational diabetes screening was carried out in 46 patients, and was normal in 31, pathological in 15 and 2 others discovered late during hospitalisation.
- Screening for trisomy 21 was carried out in 34% of cases and 1 amniocentesis was proposed for a single woman in our study with a 46XY karyotype.
- Streptococcus was detected by vaginal sampling between 34 and 38 weeks' amenorrhoea in 54% of cases.

3. Type of pregnancy

there were 48 mono-fetal pregnancies and 2 twin pregnancies

4. Pregnancy-related diseases

In our study, the following gravidic and adnexal pathologies occurred in primiparous women:

- Gestational diabetes: 34% of cases
- Pregnancy toxicity is 8%.
- Oligohydramnios (6%)
- Hydramnios, which accounts for 2% of the total

MFIU	**2%**
Prolonged pregnancy	**12%**
RPM	**14%**
Placenta previa	**2%**
MAP	**10%**

Table 9: Complications encountered during pregnancy

V. progress of labour and mode of delivery

1. The term of delivery

for deliveries before 34 days' gestation, these took place at 29 days' gestation +2 days, 28 days' gestation and 30 days' gestation +5 days.

Term	Percentage
< 34SA	6%

[34-36[	2%
[36-37[	2%
[37-41[	84%
<41SA	6%

Table 10: Term of delivery

2. How the work was carried out

2.1 Start of work

The onset of labour was spontaneous in 21 elderly primiparous women, i.e. 42%.

Artificial labour was necessary in 2 primiparous women (4%).

A planned cesarean section was performed in 27 of our elderly patients (4%) .

2.2 hard work

We cannot be sure of the exact duration of the work, as we often have little information about the exact timing of the period, but we can estimate it approximately.

We have summarised our results for our mothers in the figure below:

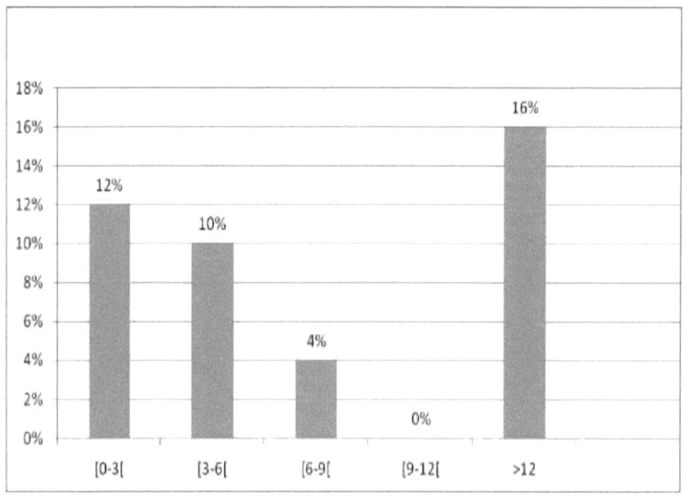

Figure 3: length of labour in older primiparous women,

2.3 Labour abnormalities

The work process was pathological in 10% of cases in the study population;

The various anomalies encountered during the work are summarised in the table below:

Anomalies	Number	%
Mechanical dystocia	4	**8%**
Dynamic dystocia	1	**2%**

Table 10: labour abnormality in primiparous women

3. Delivery method

In 16% of our patients, the mode of delivery was vaginal rather than instrumental.

Cesarean section was indicated in 84% of cases, of which 30% were urgent and 54% scheduled.

Indication	Number	%
Acute freight suffering	7	47%
Mechanical dystocia	4	27%
Prematurity and seat presentation	2	13%
Dynamic dystocia	1	7%
RPM+48H	1	7%
Procidence of cord	0	0%

Table 11: Indications for emergency cesarean section

Indication	Number	%
Advance maternal age	10	37%
Presentation	5	19%
Previous myomectomy	3	11%
Unbalanced diabetes	3	11%
Frank macrosomia	2	7%
Pre-eclampsia	2	7%
Gestational diabetes + pre-eclampsia	1	4%
Twin pregnancies	1	4%

+evanescence of J1

Table 12: Indications for prophylactic cesarean section

VI. Layer sequences

Our study shows an average hospital stay after delivery of 47 hours, with extremes of 24 and 72 hours.

No complications or maternal deaths were recorded during the study period.

- Deliverance and bleeding:

We observed a significant increase in artificial delivery in our study (84%). In our study, there were no cases of bleeding after delivery.

VII. the new age of the primipara

1. Birth weight

The average is 3188.6 (extremes 4400g and 100g).

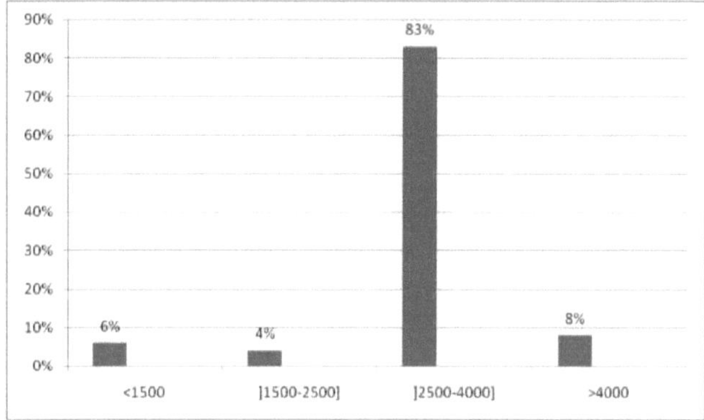

Figure 5 Birth weight of newborns from older primiparous mothers

2. APGAR score at birth

APGAR	1 minute to life		Only 5 minutes away r a 10 min			
	Number	%	Number	%	Number	%
6	1	2%	0	0%	0	0%
7	1	2%	0	0%	0	0%
8	7	13%	1	2%	1	2%
9	43	83%	10	19%	0	0%

10	0	0%	40	77%	49	94%

Table 13: APGAR score at birth of newborns from older primiparous mothers

3. Neonatal morbidity

	Number	%
Premature	5	10%
RCUI	1	2%
Macrosomia	2	4%
Neonatal mortality	1	2%

Table 14: Morbidity

4.transfer to the neonatology department

28% of newborn babies born to elderly primiparous mothers were admitted to the neonatology department

4 Discussion

I. Epidemiology

1. Definition and frequency :

1.1 Definition :

Older primiparous women are defined as women who have had their first child at an age of thirty-five or over.

The term late pregnancy applies to any pregnancy occurring after the age of 35 or even after the age of 40 (2).

In our study, we used the age limit of 38 years, which appears to be increasingly used to define an older primipara.

1.2 Frequency :

In 1984, in most Western countries, first births at the age of 40 or over represented less than 0.5% of all first births. In 2014, they represented around 2% or more in most Western countries, and 4.5% and 4.7% respectively in Spain and Italy (5). A more marked increase in 2019 in the French population, with 24.3% of births to first-time mothers aged over 40(6), which means that the phenomenon of pregnancies after the age of 35 is increasing with the years.

In Tunisia, a study of the frequency of parturients at extreme ages according to age group by K Ben Salem et al(22) showed that the 35 and over age group experienced a statistically significant increase in fagon (14.7 to 17.7%).

Another retrospective comparative case-control study conducted in the obstetric gynaecology department of the Monji Slim Hospital in La Marsa, Tunisia, over a period from 1[ere] January 2018 to 31 December 2019 showed that 280 parturients aged 40 and over were hospitalized in the department and 227/5062 deliveries, i.e. 4.4% of all deliveries managed (7).

In our study, we noted 50 primiparous women aged 38 and over out of a total of 8,548 deliveries, representing a frequency of 0.58%.

The confluence of a number of social and demographic trends in recent decades has led to an increase in the number of women becoming pregnant at a relatively early age in their reproductive lives, particularly primiparous women.

2. Breakdown by age :

The average age of our patients was 40 + 2.33 years, with extremes ranging from 38 to 47 years.

This varies from one series to another, depending on the age group chosen, and is explained by the socio-cultural differences that exist between populations.

3. Breakdown by profession :

One of the causes of late primiparity seems to be the woman's desire to achieve her professional goals before having a child.

In our series, 62% of older primiparous dams had a professional activity.

Women's education and training have made significant progress in Tunisia over the last half-century. Young women

Tunisian women are better educated than their mothers(8).

In today's society, women are no longer confined to the role of housewife, and the number of working women is increasing: in 2021, 28.2% of the working population in Tunisia will be women, compared with 23.1% in 1990(9).

11. Causes of late primiparitis

Pregnancy plans are very often postponed until at least the end of studies, and increasingly until after the acquisition of a stable job, a home and a stable relationship.

We need to make a distinction here between primiparous women who voluntarily postpone the age of their first pregnancy, and those who do so involuntarily because they are affected by treated infertility.

In the course of our work, we found that late marriage, sterility and spontaneous abortion dominate the causes of late primiparity.

1. Late marriage :

In the past, women married at an early age, but nowadays they are getting married later and later. The age at first marriage has increased significantly in Tunisia over the course of the 20th century. According to a study by Zahia Ouadah-Bedidi et al, published in 2012 and based on survey data and marriages registered at the civil registry office, the age at first marriage for women rose from 24 in 1970 to over 28 in 1990, stabilising at around 30 in the last decade

(10), the change in a woman's cultural, educational and economic status may be the cause of a delayed plan to marry.

Also, the economic conditions of a couple are often better after the age of 38 because of a longer working life and therefore the regular accumulation of capital; this leads to the decision to marry late; which represents 26% of our older primiparous women, our results are lower than those observed in the series by H. Khairi which mentioned 77% of cases (11). Nowadays, women want to find the right father, so they take their time.

2. Abortions :

Spontaneous abortion is one of the causes of late primiparity, which accounts for 42% of our elderly primiparous women.

In the series by S.Houda et al Jaccr Africa 2021 (7), ongoing abortions and terminated pregnancies were found in 10.6% of cases.

In the general population, the risk of miscarriage is 1 in 5 pregnancies. This risk increases with maternal age and, from the age of 40, is estimated to be 1 in 3 pregnancies(12).

All the authors therefore agree that the percentage of spontaneous miscarriages increases with maternal age, irrespective of parity.

3. Infertility:

Concerning antecedents of infertility, we found 32% of our older primiparous women, of whom 8 pregnancies were obtained by MAP.

In the jazia series (11), 14% of primiparous women were being monitored for infertility.

The proportion of women aged 40 and over who had recourse to MAP was around 12% in 2012, according to FIV.Fr data (13).

We saw earlier that fertility and fecundity fall with age (12,14), yet 64% of our primiparous women over 38 became pregnant spontaneously.

4. Other causes :

Improved and more widespread contraceptive techniques have also made it possible to control fertility. There is now a long period between first intercourse and the first child.

A change of spouse appears to be another cause of late procreation. Our study did not include a change of spouse.

III. Pathologies prior to pregnancy:

Although motherhood at this age remains, in the majority of cases, a happy motherhood, it is important to highlight certain risks in order to pay particular attention to them as a professional.

1. Medical pathologies:

The literature is unanimous in stating that pre-existing pathologies are all more common in women aged 40 and over: hypertension, fibroids, diabetes, heart problems and thyroid dysfunction (15). In our study, 22% of older primiparous women had at least one medical condition in their antecedents, of which 4% were diabetic and 2% hypertensive. Contrary to some data in the international literature, the frequency of chronic maternal diseases preexisting during pregnancy, such as preexisting chronic arterial hypertension which is observed in 1 to 5% of pregnancies (16), preexisting diabetes occurs in > 6% of pregnancies (17)...

Our results were comparable to those described in the Tunisian literature, In the series by ben jazia (11) 11.8% of primiparous women had at least one medical condition in their antecedents.

2. Surgical pathologies :

As women age, they are more exposed to surgical conditions.

In our study, 18% of elderly primiparous women had a surgical antecedent. Our results were in line with the literature. However, our frequency was higher.

3. Gyneco-obstetric pathologies:

In our series, we noted an increase in the frequency of spontaneous abortions (42%), uterine fibroids (8%) and ovarian cysts (6%) in older primiparous women. Miscarriages and fibroids were the 2 most frequently noted gynaeco-obstetric antecedents in both our series and that of ben jazia (11).

The rate of spontaneous miscarriage more than doubles with age: from 11.7%

between the ages of 30 and 34, it rises to 33.8% over the age of 40 (18).

In the literature, 20% of women over 35 have uterine fibroids (17).

IV. Pregnancy:

1. Pregnancy mode:

In our series, the majority of pregnancies were spontaneous, i.e. 64% of primiparous women, similar to that described in other Tunisian series, citing Jazia (11) who mentioned 93.6% of spontaneous pregnancies in primiparous women.

Dildy et al (19) carried out a study of 126,500 births over 10 years. They found 79 pregnancies in mothers aged 45 and over, with only three resulting from MAP.

Spontaneous pregnancy is still possible after the age of 40, but women should not be led to believe that it is easy. In fact, for some women it has been difficult to achieve 1, despite sometimes having recourse to MAP. Before talking about sterility, we need to look at fecundity, which is the probability of conceiving at each cycle. The age of the mother, the sexuality of the coup le and the duration of infecundity must all be taken into account. Pregnancy seems to be a genuine programmed choice at a given point in their lives.

2. Pregnancy follow-up :

Pregnancy is a period of great psychological upheaval for pregnant women, whatever their maternal age. Pregnancy is a life experience full of contradictory emotions: hope, happiness, fear and anxiety.

The context of achieving a late pregnancy in a primiparous woman after the age of 40 is not experienced in the same way as a pregnancy in a young primiparous woman. These pregnancies may be obtained after several experiences of abortion or failed attempts at medically assisted procreation. Couples are also subject to social stress from those around them. However, families can put particular pressure on women.

Because of the age of the parturient and the fragility of the product of conception, pregnancies in elderly primiparous women require close maternal-fetal monitoring throughout the pregnancy and during labour.

The aim of this monitoring is to reduce pregnancy complications and maintain a prognosis for pregnancy similar to that seen in young primiparous dams.

We note that the percentage of correctly monitored pregnancies (prenatal consultations) is around 92% in our study population.

This notion has been noted by most authors, including S Houda et al.(7) during the study period, 76% of patients over 40 years of age had at least 2 antenatal consultations.

Almost all studies show an increase in the frequency of gestational diabetes in late pregnancies.

In our study, 46 patients were screened for gestational diabetes. The result was normal in 31 of them. It was pathological in 15 patients, i.e. 30% of diabetics, 4% of whom had diabetes.

The prevalence of gestational diabetes was 3 times higher overall in older women, according to various series published in the literature (20,21).

Given the high incidence of this condition in primiparous women aged 40 and over, these women should be systematically screened in the first trimester, especially if there is a family or personal predisposition. An oral induced hyperglycaemia should therefore be carried out between 24 and 28 weeks' amenorrhoea, to make the diagnosis.

3. Type of pregnancy :

In our study, we found 48 singleton pregnancies and 2 twin pregnancies. However, we note that there is a trend towards an increase in this frequency, which has tripled since the study by ben jazia (11), who found 6 gemellar pregnancies.

According to data from the sentinel network of the association of users of computerised records in paediatrics, obstetrics and gynaecology, the rate of multiple pregnancies between the ages of 40 and 50 is 1.79%, compared with 1.55% in the 20-35 age group. However, while there has been a slight increase in the rate of twin pregnancies in women over 40, the use of MAP must be taken into account. Older women are more likely to have recourse to these techniques. In this case, two or more embryos are frequently implanted.

4. Pregnancy-related diseases:

Maternal age is a determining factor in maternal and infant morbidity and mortality (23,24,25).

All authors agree that pregnancies at the extreme ages of reproductive life (19 years, 35 years) expose women to sometimes very serious complications (toxemia, eclampsia, mechanical dystonia, diabetes, postpartum haemorrhage) (26) and sometimes unfavourable outcomes (low birth weight babies, stillbirths, prematurity, AFS....) (27,28).

The most common pathology was gestational diabetes, with 34% of primiparous women over 38 years of age. Our values are similar to those found by Gilbert et al (29). In Tunisia, too, gestational diabetes was more frequently observed in the population aged 40 and over, according to the study by F Zhioua et al (30).

In second place is arterial hypertension, which accounts for 6% of our older primiparous dams. Gilbert observed only 5.4% of hypertension in primiparous women over 40 (29).

the frequency of gestational hypertension was increased in the majority of series (20,31).

For pregnancy toxemia, our study found 8% of cases, which is very low compared to other studies (7,29).

Eclampsia is the first complication to be feared in toxic patients, and is becoming increasingly rare. Our series notes only one case. This could be explained by better monitoring and prevention of complications of pregnancy-related toxemia.

Obesity or excessive weight gain before or during pregnancy is a risk factor for complications in women aged 35 and over, particularly gestational diabetes.

In our series, 54% of primiparous women were obese.

The association between maternal age and obesity has been cited by some authors as justification for very early screening for unknown diabetes prior to pregnancy and fasting blood glucose tests in the first trimester(32).

As part of standard pregnancy monitoring, it is also important to provide all older primiparous women with health and diet advice, especially if they are overweight or obese.

5. Complications during pregnancy :

The number of patients in this study was too small to study maternal and perinatal complications, as well as maternal mortality (no maternal deaths observed).

J With regard to the threat of premature delivery, our study found that 10% of pregnancies were affected. Our values are close to those found by Luke and Ziadeh (42, 43).

J also observed 14% premature rupture of the membranes. Whereas F Zhioua et al (30) premature rupture of the water sac was observed in 25.7% of cases in the group of women aged 40 and over.premature rupture of the membranes remains high in women of advanced age for the majority of authors (7,33).

J For over term, our percentage is 12% in the study population, close to that of KUDDER (11) who found it in 10% of old primiparous women.

J Placenta previa is a rare pathology. In our series we observed only one case, i.e. 2% of all our primiparous women.

Several studies (20, 31) report similar frequencies, while Gilbert et al (29) and Ananth (34) respectively found an 8-fold and 9-fold relative risk of placenta previa in primiparous women aged 40 and over compared with younger women.

J For retro-placental hematoma, our series, like that of other authors (32,7), found no cases. Opinions are much more divergent concerning placental abruption. For some, age is not a risk factor, but rather the associated parity and hypertension which pose a problem. Others conclude that there is no correlation between age and the occurrence of this type of pathology. (29)

So primiparity after the age of 38 does constitute a risk for the onset of obstetric pathologies. However, late pregnancies should not be demonised, as most will have a favourable outcome. Nevertheless, it is important to remain vigilant in the face of existing risks and to monitor these pregnancies closely.

v. progress of labour and mode of delivery :

1. The term of delivery :

Although the majority of deliveries took place between 37 and 41 weeks' gestation (84%), 6% of births took place after the theoretical date of 41 weeks' gestation. Thus, the frequency of onset in these women could be explained by the fact that pregnancies are often prolonged beyond 41SAS and that a pathology may be associated. In addition, the protocols mean that we tend to be more interventionist from a certain term onwards. From 41 weeks' gestation onwards, the pregnancy must be closely monitored to ensure the well-being of the fetus. It will be necessary to check whether or not obstetric conditions are favourable to induction. To do this, the Bishop score is calculated.

2. Work in progress:

2.1.Start of work:

In our study, labour was induced in 4% of primiparous women, a lower rate than that reported by PRYSAK (35) who found 17.2% of cases.

The indications for labour induction in our elderly primiparous women were dominated by PMR and prolonged pregnancy.

Thus 54% of our older primiparous women had a caesarean section before going into labour. According to the national antenatal survey (2010), this rate is higher in primiparous women aged over 40 than in the general population (48% versus 33.5%) (36).

In 42% of cases, labour in our older primiparous women was spontaneous, but our figures are still very low compared with others such as PRYSAK (35) who cite 74% of cases.

2.2.Working hours :

The end of labour is always precise, as it is the exact time of birth, but the beginning is vague. It is accepted that labour begins with the onset of regular, painful contractions, which is subjective and imprecise because it is estimated retrospectively.

In our study, we noted that 16% of older primiparous women had a duration of labour in excess of 12 hours. This notion is noted by most authors, REMELTS (11), studying the mean duration of deliveries in 5915 primiparous women, established an ascending curve with age.

2.3.Labour abnormalities :

Labour in the elderly primipara is not only slow, but also fraught with complications. In our work, we reported complications during labour, namely dynamic dystocia and mechanical dystocia, with rates of 2% and 8% respectively.

The physiological basis of this frequency of labour anomalies in older primiparous women is unclear. However, authors have blamed uterine hypoplasia, reduced functional value and uterine muscle fibre invaded by fibrosis with age, and the greater frequency of uterine fibroids (7, 22, 37).

3. Delivery method :

3.1.Cesarean delivery :

In our older primiparous women, 54% of cesarean sections were performed before the onset of labour. The indications were essentially advanced maternal age in 10 patients, i.e. 37% of prophylactic cesarean sections, while some of the cesarean sections could also be explained by an increase in seat presentations, 5 older primiparous women, i.e. 19% of cases, and 3 patients, i.e. 11%, benefited from a prophylactic cesarean section for a history of myomectomy.

The more frequent recourse to a planned cesarean section in older women has been observed by all authors in all countries (22,37,38). It is also possible that parental anxiety plays a role, as this may influence the obstetrician's approach.

However, we can question the wisdom of such a practice, which leads to an increase in postoperative maternal morbidity, especially as this population of women has additional risk factors compared with young mothers (22, 35).

Finally, from a psychological point of view, some authors consider that practitioners find cesarean sections "easier" and that patients are more "demanding" of this type of delivery. (7)

30% of cesarean sections were performed during labour. SFA was the first indication for emergency cesarean section in our primiparous women with a rate of 47%, mechanical dystocia represented 27% of indications for emergency cesarean section, and prematurity was indicated in 2 elderly primiparous women, i.e. 13% of indications for cesarean section during labour. This result is close to that of F ZHIOUA (30).

There is a higher risk of caesarean section during labour in older women, a fact observed by the majority of authors (30).

The increase in obstetric pathologies is leading to greater vigilance over the progress of labour, and we can assume that obstetricians will be quicker to decide to perform a caesarean section at the slightest abnormality, given the increased risks associated with these pregnancies.

Even if the cesarean section rate is high, it is important to bear in mind that cesarean section is not the preferred mode of delivery for these women. In fact, "elderly primiparous" should not be a systematic indication. However, this was the case in my study. The indication should therefore be based on the patient's history and any complications in the current pregnancy.

3.2.Normal delivery :

In our study, the mode of vaginal delivery was 16%, of which 16% was non-instrumental and 0% instrumental. This rate is lower than those quoted by most authors (11).

VI. Layer sequence :

1. Deliverance and bleeding:

We observed a significant increase in artificial delivery in our study (84%), as we had a much higher rate of cesarean section in this population, and consequently artificial delivery during the operation.

In our study, there were no cases of delivery haemorrhage.

2. Length of stay :

In our series, the average length of hospital stay was 47 hours, with extremes ranging from 24 hours to 72 hours, whatever the route of delivery.

In ben jazia's series (11) this duration was 2.8 days.

3. Maternal mortality :

By definition, maternal mortality includes any "death occurring during pregnancy or within 42 days of its end, whatever its duration or location, from any cause related to or aggravated by pregnancy or the care it may have prompted, with the exception of accidental or fortuitous causes". According to INSERM data for the period 1998 to 2000, the risk of maternal death is 3 times higher in women aged 35 to 50, compared with younger women. It is most frequent after the age of 45. In fact, women over 45 are 15 times more likely to die during pregnancy and in the post-partum period. These deaths are mainly due to haemorrhage, hypertension-related accidents and thromboembolic pathologies(22).

In our study, there were no cases of maternal death.

4. Maternal morbidity:

Concerning post-partum pathologies. The results were more difficult to obtain, as the diagnosis was not always precise.

According to the literature, anxiety and baby-blues following childbirth are prevalent in mothers aged 40 and over. However, we did not study this criterion in our study due to the difficulty of collecting this data.

VII. newborn in the elderly primipara :

1. Birth weight :

Many authors believe that the weight of newborns born to older primiparous women is lower than normal, due to maternal age and antecedents.

However, in our study, the average weight was 3188.6 692g (extremes: 4400g and 1000g) in older primiparous mothers. However, if we compare full-term newborns, the average weight is closer to the national average of around 3200g.

This value is comparable to that of ben jazia (11) who, in his study, found an average birth weight of 3180g.

Advanced maternal age is thought to be involved in a greater frequency of low birth weight or, conversely, macrosomia. This may be explained by poor placental perfusion of the older uterus and/or gravid vasculo-renal pathology in the case of hypotrophy, and by diabetes in the case of macrosomia.

2. APGAR score at birth :

We studied the APGAR score of neonates born to older primiparous women at 1, 5 and 10 minutes of life. We compared our results with those in the literature. Most authors emphasise the high risk of heart failure in older primiparous women, with many noting a lower APGAR score in newborns of primiparous women than in other newborns.

In our series we found 2% of newborns with a one-minute APGAR score of 6, 2% with a score of 7, 13% with a score of 8, and 83% with a score of 9.

Jahromi et al (31) found an Apgar <7 in 17.3% of patients aged over 40 compared with 11% in the control group and the difference was significant. Bianco (20) found no significant difference with a rate of 0.9%.

3. Neonatal morbidity and mortality:

3.1.Freight mortality :

Mortality in recent studies such as those by Luke and Gilbert ranges from 0.4 to 0.7% (29). In our study, one case of fretal death in utero was found, bringing the mortality rate to 2%, but given the small sample size of our study, we cannot draw any significant conclusions on this subject.

The loss of a baby is a disappointment for the family, particularly for the elderly primiparous woman who wants the baby. The midwife must therefore remain alert to the risk of fretal death. Clinically, the active movements of the fretus should be carefully monitored. The well-being of the fetus can also be assessed by recording the fetal heart rate and using a Manning score.

1.2.Neonatal morbidity :

We found 2 macrosomic newborns, despite more frequent gestational diabetes. We can therefore assume that diabetes monitoring and balance were correct;

The perinatal complications studied were intrauterine growth retardation (IUGR) defined by a birth weight below the fifth percentile, according to the Lubchenco curves (39), and premature delivery before 37 weeks' gestation, of which 2% and 10% respectively were noted.

We did not observe any congenital malformations in the newborns of the mothers in our study. However, our study only included live births, whereas most congenital anomalies are detected in-utero and may lead to an indication for medical termination of pregnancy.

4. Transfer to the Neonatology Department:

Transfers to intensive care units were significantly more frequent (28%). This confirms the data provided by W. Gilbert (29). On the other hand, the vast majority of children had a relatively good APGAR at birth.

We can hypothesise that these more frequent transfers are induced by increased prematurity and a greater number of maternal and fetal pathologies, and not by the maternal page itself.

5 Recommendations

It's important to remember that it's our duty to provide clear, appropriate information to all our patients. What's more, patients who consult a midwife after the age of 38 because they want to become pregnant legitimately want to be provided with adequate information about the basics of pregnancy monitoring and the midwife's skills in this area.

The midwife's skills in pregnancy monitoring:

Midwives practise a medical profession with defined competence, i.e. the Public Health Code (CSP) has determined their field of intervention, which is devoted to physiology and also includes the practice of acts necessary for the diagnosis of pathology.

The midwife is therefore fully autonomous in monitoring normal pregnancies, from notification to the postnatal consultation. (40,41)

Midwives are involved in primary health care in the same way as general practitioners and medical gynaecologists, which is why they are responsible for assessing women's risk levels and referring them to gynaecologists and obstetricians if risk factors are present or appear.

The basics of monitoring a late pregnancy

pregnancy :

It is important for the midwife to carry out an accurate and complete history-taking on these primiparous women. This will enable her to assess the risks incurred by the patient with regard to her past history. More careful monitoring of the pregnancy should be considered for certain pathologies. Specific examinations and treatment may be necessary, as well as changing or stopping current treatment.

Ultrasound monitoring should be meticulous, with one scan per trimester, paying particular attention to signs of abnormality or malformation, and to biometry. In the event of maternal or fetal pathology, more intensive monitoring should be instituted (40).

Genetic counselling addresses the prognosis for the current pregnancy. The doctor will be able to reduce the uncertainty and doubt that cause anxiety in patients. (40)

As for serum markers, the future would be a study based on the joint measurement of nuchal translucency, HCG and a placental protein, PAPP-A.

This earlier screening has a reliability rate of around 80% for trisomy 21.

It is not very practical but should be developed in women at risk of chromosomal abnormalities. However, in cases of high risk, amniocentesis will remain the test of choice. (40)

The possibility of antenatal diagnosis should be discussed with patients at the start of their pregnancy. Some, because of religious or personal convictions, do not wish to enter into a "care" system aimed at discovering and eliminating babies with chromosomal abnormalities. Others cannot bear the risk of bringing a child with Down's syndrome into the world and want antenatal diagnosis to be

carried out, even if this means taking an invasive sample. (40)
In addition, late amniocentesis can always be carried out if necessary. This examination will continue to be offered as a matter of course, but the benefits and risks must be weighed up.
The midwife must therefore remain alert to the risk of fretal death. Clinically, the active movements of the fretus should be carefully monitored. Fetal well-being can also be assessed by recording the fetal heart rate and using a Manning score.
In view of the high incidence of gestational diabetes in primiparous women aged 40, systematic screening of these women between 24 and 28 weeks of amenorrhoea should be considered (40).
In addition, it seems essential to inform the patient of the risk of threatened premature delivery, so that she can recognise the signs. She should be encouraged to seek medical advice if she experiences painful uterine contractions, bleeding or febrile episodes that may indicate infection, and should be advised to rest more. During consultations, the midwife will carry out a urine test using a strip to check the leucocyte count. A cytobacteriological examination of the urine will be prescribed in the event of a pathological result or any other abnormal sign. A vaginal swab should also be taken to check for vaginal infection: this is carried out systematically between 32 and 36 weeks' gestation (40).
Blood pressure, albuminuria and redemas should be monitored systematically at each monthly consultation. If there are additional risk factors, a midwife or the PMI midwife can be called in for closer monitoring. The patient should also be informed of the signs that should attract her attention: severe swelling of the ankles, hands or face, rapid weight gain, headaches, tinnitus, phosphenes or stomach pain (40).
During labour, you must be vigilant for abnormalities in the fetal heart rate.
This does not mean that the child should be extracted straight away, as various tests can be carried out in the event of a suspicious fretal heart rhythm.

For example, labour monitoring in a 40-year-old primipara is no different from that of a younger woman (40).

6 Conclusion

First pregnancies after the age of 38 are now a real phenomenon in society, and one that has been steadily increasing over the last few years. Nowadays, women's health is generally better, thanks to health and hygiene habits that are much better than they were in the middle of the twentieth century. But in the context of childbearing, there is ample evidence that advanced age is a major risk factor. Leaving aside the reduction in fertility and the consequent difficulties in conceiving.

The aim of our study was to observe the maternal and freight complications induced by maternal age on the course of pregnancy, delivery and the neonatal state. The study confirmed that maternal age was responsible for the appearance of numerous obstetric complications: gestational hypertension, gestational diabetes and premature rupture of membranes, the incidence of which increases with age. In addition, the delivery of patients aged 38 and over may be complicated by cesarean section, delivery haemorrhage and hypotrophic infants, with neonatal adjustment sometimes more difficult. When the patient is admitted to the delivery room, it is important to be aware of these possible risks, so that the obstetric team can be as prepared as possible and anticipate any abnormalities in labour and delivery. The same applies to possible postpartum complications. Pregnancies after the age of 38 must therefore be monitored with particular care. This context demands rigorous monitoring, by a midwife in the case of a normal pregnancy, or by a gynaecologist-obstetrician for complicated pregnancies. However, the midwife is rarely involved in monitoring late pregnancies, a fact that is mainly down to the patient's choice. This choice is linked to the patient's antecedents or her own perceptions of a late pregnancy, the influence that the opinions of her family and friends and society in general may have on this type of pregnancy, and finally a lack of knowledge about the competence of a midwife to monitor a late pregnancy. However, given that the cost of monitoring a pregnancy is lower for a midwife than for an obstetrician, it would be appropriate to raise public awareness of the skills of midwives in general, and particularly in pregnancies considered to be at risk.

However, it is our role as healthcare professionals to inform these women, who are over 38 and who want to become mothers for the first time, of the risks they run. It is essential to monitor and support these couples to ensure that they receive the best possible care, so that any complications can be detected.

Reference

(1) WHO. Antenatal care.
http://www.who.int/reproductivehealth/publications/maternal_perinatal_health/ANC_infographics/en/ . 2013; [accessed 22 Dec 2017].

(2) mosby's medical dictionary 8th edition maryland heights Eservier E-BOOK

(3) -Ballo AB. Grossesse et accouchement chez la primipare âge dans les services de gynecologie-obstetrique de l'hopital Gabriel Toure et du Point <<G>>These BAMAKO 2004-2005. n°136

(4) Belaisch-Allart J. , Grosssese et acouchement apres 40 ans.EMC (Elsevier Masson SAS,Paris),Gynecologie et Obstetrique 5-016-B-10,2008.

(5) Beaujouan, Eva, and Tomas Sobotka. " Les maternites tardives : de plus en plus frequentes dans les pays developpes ", Population & Societes, 2019 vol. 562, p2

(6) Insee, census surveys for 2019 and 2020 (main surveys) Available at: https://www.insee.fr/fr/statistiques/6019324#titre-bloc- 19

(7) S Houda et al. Jacc Africa 2021
https://jaccrafrica.com/gallery/001l01020121v4n4%20s%20houda%20et%20al.%20grossesse%20age%20avance.pdf

(8) Women and employment in Tunisia
https://www.etf.europa.eu/sites/default/files/im/B68A324BD9A09110C12578F8004D957FWomen%20%26%20work TunisiaEN.pdf

(9) Female employment rate in Tunisia
https://donnees.banquemondiale.org/indicator/SL.TLF.CACT.FM.NE.ZS?locations=TN

(10) Tunisia late marriage: https://fr.allafrica.com/stories/201303252022.html

(11) Ben jazia M. grossesse et accouchement chez lez primipare agees these de Medecine , Monastir 2000.
https://www.sciencedirect.com/journal/annales-francaises-danesthesie-et-de- resuscitation

(12) https://www.chusj.org/fr/soins-services/C/complications-de- pregnancy/complications-mother/Complications/miscarriages-abortions-repeat

(13) https://www.fiv.fr/statistiques-fiv/

(14) https://www.latunisiemedicale.com/pdf/VOL 88 N01 n6 REF1-4.pdf

(15) Joseph K, Allen A, Dodds L, Turner L et al. The perinatal effect of delayed childbearing.Obstet Gynecol 2005;105:1410-1418.

(16) Hypertensions et grossesse : aspects epidemiologiques, definitionHypertension during pregnancy: Epidemiology, definition

https://www.sciencedirect.com/science/article/abs/pii/S0755498216301348

(17) https://www.msdmanuals.com/fr/professional/gyn%C3%A9cologie-et-obst%C3%A9tric/pregnancy-%C3%A0-high-risk/risk-factors-of-complications-depending-on-pregnancy

(18) BELAISCH-ALLART J., Grossesses tardives : apres 35 ans, les femmes doivent consulter, Le quotidien du medecin, n°8419, 16 September 2008

(19) DILDY (GA), JACKSON (GM), FA VERS (GK) et al. Very advanced matemal age :pregnancy after age 45. Obstet. Gynecol, 1 996, 1 75 : 668-74.

(20) Bianco A, Stone J, Lynch L,Lapinski R, Berkowitz G, Bekowitz R , pregnancy autcome at age 40 and older https://pubmed.ncbi.nlm.nih.gov/8649698/

(21) Vercellini P , Zuliani G, Rpgnoni MT, Trespidi L, OldaniL, Cardinal A. pregnancy at 40 and over

(22) Kamel Ben Salem, Sana El Mhamdi, Imen Ben Amor, Asma Sriha, Mondher Letaief, Mohamed Soussi Soltani Epidemiological And Chronological Profile Of The Parturientes In The Extreme Ages In The Monastir Region Between 1994 And 2003

(23) Treffers PE. Teenage pregnancy, a worldwide problem. Ned Tijdschr Geneeskd 2003; 22:2320-5.

(24) Heffner LJ, Elkin E, Fretts RC. Impact of labor induction, gestational age and maternal age on cesarean delivery rates. Obstet.Gynecol 2003; 102:287-293.

(25) Tabcharoen C, Pinjaroen S, Suwanrath C, Krisanapan O. Pregnancy outcome after age 40 and risk of low birth weight. J Obstet Gynaecol 2009; 29:378-83.

(26) Ozalp S, Mete TH, Sener T, Yazan S, Keskin AE. Health risks for early[2] 19 and late ? 35 year childbearing. Arch Gynecol Obstet 2003; 268: 172-174.

(27) Huang L, Sauve R, Birkett N, Fergusson D, van Walraven C. Maternal age and risk of stillbirth: a systematic review. CMAJ 2008; 178:165-72.

(28) Kumar A, Singh T, Basu S, Pandey S, Bhargava V. Outcome of teenage pregnancy. Indian J Pediatr 2007; 74:927-31.

(29) W.GILBERT, TS NESBITT, B.DANIELSON, Childbearing beyond age 40: pregnancy outcome in 24032 cases, Obstet Gynecol n°93, 1999; p. 9-14

(30) Asma Jnifen, Anis Fadhlaoui, Anis Chaker, Fethi Zhioua Particularites de la grossesse et de l'accouchement chez la femme de 40 ans et plus : A propos de 300 cas La tunisie Medicale - 2010 ; Vol 88 (n°011) : 829 - 833

(31) Jahromi BN, Hussein Z. Pregnancy outcome at maternal age 40 and older .Taiwan J Obstet Gynecol 2008; 47 -3.

(32) Marie Aussedat. The role of the midwife in monitoring the pregnancies of elderly primiparous women. Medecine humaine et pathologie. 2011. ffhal-01881956

(33) Audipot B,Arnaud F,childbirth and complications after 35 years .J Gynecol REs

(34) Ananth CV, Wilcox AJ, Avitz DA et al. Effect of maternal age and parity on the risk of uteroplacental bleeding disorders in pregnancy. Obstet Gynecol1996; 88: 5116.

(35) PRYSAK (M), LORENTZ (RP), KISL Y (A). Pregnancy outcome in nulliparous women 35 years and older. Obstet. Gynecol. , 1 995, 85 : 65-70.

(36) Enquete nationale prenatale 2010 tableaux des chiffres .Les naissances en 2010 et leur evolution depuis 2003 .Paris Elsevier 2011.

(37) Schoen C, Rosen T. Maternal and perinatal risks for women over 44--a review. Maturitas 2009; 64:109-13.

(38) Santos GH, Martins Mda G, Sousa Mda S, Batalha Sde J. Impact of maternal age on perinatal outcomes and mode of delivery. Rev Bras Ginecol Obstet 2009; 31:326-34.

(39) https://www.audipog.net/pdf/seminaires/seminaire 2008/pres06 audipog.p df

(40) www.atds.org.tn > Public Health Code 4

(41)DRAWING UP JOB AND SKILLS REFERENCES FOR MIDWIVES IN TUNISIA https://tunisia.unfpa.org/sites/default/files/pub-pdf/cadre pedagogique et methodologique -conceptionvalidee 20062022.pdf

(42)Luke B,Brown M. Elevated risks of pregnancy complications and adverse outcome with increasing maternal age .Hum reprod 2007 ;22 :1264-72

(43)Ziadeh S,Yahaya A.Pregnancy outcome at age 40 and older .arch Gynecol obstet2001

(44)

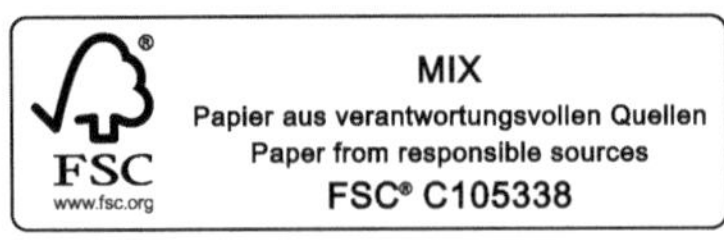

Printed by Books on Demand GmbH, Norderstedt / Germany